MW00872748

Creating the French Metabolism

Eat, Drink, and be Beautiful

Kelley Pom

Illustrations by Regan James

Copyright © 2019 Kelley Pom

All rights reserved.

ISBN: 9781082089718

DEDICATION

To Jeff, Chris, and Regan, whose love and support make it possible for me to do anything, and who make my life So Freaking French.

CONTENTS

Acknowledgments   i

1   Why Can't you Just Eat ... Food?   1

2   I Should Have Been Fat   5

3   Fact vs. ... *Fact?* The Problem with Diets   12

4   A French Frame of Mind   19

5   The First Factor – Your Relationship with Food   23

6   The Second Factor – The Quality of Food you Eat   34

7   The Third Factor – Movement (A.K.A. Exercise)   44

8   Putting it All Together   49

9   If You Need to Lose Weight   54

10   Kitchen Staples, Meal Suggestions and Simple Recipes   59

11   Your Final French Metabolism Guideline   79

French Metabolism Cheat Sheet   81

What's Next?   82

ACKNOWLEDGMENTS

I'm so blessed to have so many wonderful people in my life who love me enough to make me think I could write a book. I can't begin to express my gratitude, but I'll make a feeble attempt.

First, I have to thank my husband, my editor, and my hero, Jeff Pomerantz, for rescuing me from my darkest places and whisking me away to Paris, and for laughing in all the right places.

Thank you to my daughter Regan James for the magnificent illustrations, for loving everything I write, and for being my best turtle.

Thank you to my son Chris Scoggins for the encouragement and amazing photos. You can count on me like 1-2-3 ...

I also want to thank –

Lou Pine, for stealing my daughter's heart, and taking such good care of it. Thank you for being the best son-in-law I could ever wish for.

Sarah Scoggins, for being a wonderful daughter-in-law, for being my test kitchen, and for Hector.

Jessica, Josh and Chiara, the best step-kids ever and I'm happy to be your Wicked Step-Mother.

Robin Bogan, you've had my back for over 30 years, and I love you.

Darrel and Leslie, I wouldn't even know where to start.

My beautiful LOLAs, for getting me through the rough spots.

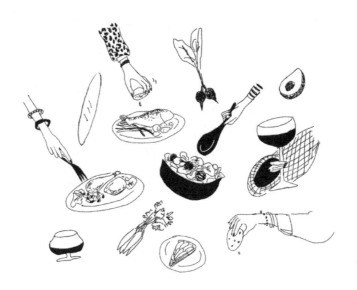

CHAPTER 1
WHY CAN'T YOU JUST EAT ... *FOOD?*

This is not a diet book. I'm not going to tell you that sugar is the devil, or that the road to hell is paved with grains.

This is the end-of-diets book, an anti-diet; a mindset, and an eating way of life.

There's no need to go looking for that *one* chapter in the book (the one you search out and read first in every diet book ... *I know*) that tells you *exactly* what to eat and what not to eat, or what to weigh or count or measure, because it isn't there. There are no rules about when you can "cheat", because how can you cheat when nothing is forbidden? (And who would you be cheating, anyway?)

What you will learn, chapter by chapter, is how to eat real food without torture, deprivation, or eliminating whole groups of food, while maintaining an optimum weight. You'll learn the reasons why you've had any difficulties in managing your weight in the past, and why it's not your fault. And you'll learn a whole new attitude toward food and eating.

Imagine maintaining your perfect size without continually denying yourself. Eating bread and enjoying a glass of wine without guilt or consequences. Never bemoaning all the *calories* you just ate.

What I'm describing is not only possible, it is the French way of life. Part of it anyway.

If you've struggled with weight, or had problems with achieving or maintaining your ideal weight, you may want to think there's something physically wrong with you that's causing your struggle. There's probably not. You might think it's all your fault, due to your lack of will-power or some other shortcoming. It probably isn't. But there are reasons, as you will soon see, and it's all within your control.

What's wrong with eating like an American?

On average, the American "eating lifestyle" results in a gain of about one to two pounds about one a year, starting as early as our mid-20's.

One or two pounds is no big deal, right? Here's the problem with that – math. That one or two pounds results in another 10 – 20 pounds of *you* every 10 years.

We've sort of gotten accustomed to the idea that people put on weight as they age. We look at the before and after photos of some of our favorite childhood celebrities, and often the first thing we notice is how much weight they've put on. And we figure yeah, well, that's what happens. But it doesn't have to.

Yes, there are a number of factors that go into why we gain weight as we age, and we'll talk about those. But the French way of eating includes balancing things out and making adjustments, so the weight doesn't have to accumulate.

If you're sort of fine with the idea of packing on an extra 20 or so pounds every 10 years for the remainder of your life, then I guess you can close the book and take a nap. But if you want to maintain an ideal weight and an active lifestyle from here on out, keep reading *s'il vous plait.*

Why learn to eat like a French woman from an American?

Have you ever had someone much more knowledgeable than you in computers try to explain something on the computer? Or had a musician explain advanced techniques and chord progressions? Or a professional dancer show you a combination of moves?

There's a little something called *The Curse of Knowledge,* and it occurs when someone with a strong understanding or background in a subject assumes you have the same understanding or background, and so over-simplifies or under-explains the subject they're trying to communicate.

I've read several well-written books by lovely French women, who will tell you, "Just do this." "Just do that." Boom, bam, you're skinny! No, I'm sorry, but we Americans need just a little more context, if you please.

Being born *extremely* American, as you'll soon see, I have *no* curse of knowledge. Everything I know, I learned the hard way.

So just think of me as your French *maman.*

Through my travels, research, observation and personal experience, I have made discoveries that unlock the "secrets" of the French metabolism. They are not secrets if you grew up in France, since it is a way of life. But just like riding a bicycle, anything can be learned. You just have to know the fundamentals.

What I'm giving you are habits and lifestyle changes that allow you to reach and maintain your desired body size without diets and deprivation. I'll show you why you've had problems maintaining your weight in the past, and why it's not entirely your fault.

If you're currently overweight, later in the book I will help you lose weight in a healthy way and in a relatively quick amount of time, without feeling tortured (yes, I know I told you I'm not going to tell you exactly *what* to eat, but I will tell you *how*.)

I will also give you a few simple, delicious food ideas to get you started on your French metabolism journey. You'll want to prepare most of your own food, as the French do, because it will be healthier and more delicious than most of the food you get from a restaurant. But don't worry, I'll make that easy too.

This book is for you if ...

- You've tried everything from paleo to vegan and can't stick with it long enough to get results, or gain back everything as soon as you stop
- You can lose weight but just can't stay at your ideal weight
- You've steadily gained a pound or two year after year (or want to avoid that)
- You're just not sure what or how to eat to maintain your "happy weight"
- You're a closet eater
- You want to be one of "those people" who can enjoy great food and not obsess about it

The guidelines in this book are simple – so simple in fact that you may not believe it. That's ok, because it's not about belief. It's all about *doing* each step until it becomes second nature, just as if you'd been born French.

Welcome, and enjoy!

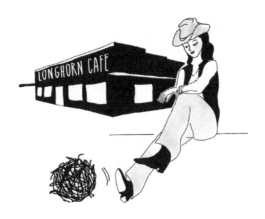

CHAPTER 2
I SHOULD HAVE BEEN FAT

It was the perfect recipe for disaster. I grew up in Texas. In the 60's and 70's. With a very overweight family. Who owned a café.

If what's wrong with all that isn't immediately evident, let me explain.

- Texas is known for many things – a slow, southern drawl; fields of corn, cotton and cattle; and country music. It is not known for its healthy way of eating. Fried chicken, chicken fried steak, fried catfish, hushpuppies, biscuits and gravy, cornbread and butter; that's home cooking in the south – and it's often served in all-you-can-eat proportions, which explains the 33% obesity rate in Texas.

- In the 60's and 70's, a lot less was known and understood about nutrition. Add to that the advent of "miracle" processed foods as more and more women entered the work force. I remember what a treat it was to have "TV dinners" and "Instant Breakfast" and things made with God-knows-what to keep them preserved in space.

  Since the introduction of these miracle foods, obesity rates in America have more than doubled from 13% in 1960 to over 30% in 2000.

- If genetics do play some slight role in obesity, I should be genetically wired to be overweight like the rest of my family. They weren't hugely obese, but they were all well down the road from what you'd call "pleasantly plump".

  However, a recent Harvard study showed that, when it comes to genetic obesity, it is the *consumption of certain foods*, such as fried foods, which interact with *genes related to obesity*. So, while there may be a link to genetics and obesity, you can control your destiny by not feeding your "fat genes".

  And boy, did my family know how to feed the fat genes!

- We owned the only café in our small town of 500 people – the Longhorn Café in Cranfills Gap, Texas. It was exactly what you might envision as a small country diner in the middle of nowhere, with red leatherette stools at the counter which were fun to spin around on until you were dizzy, and red leatherette booths with Formica-topped tables lining the walls.

  My grandfather left at around 5:00 every morning to start preparing some of the best Texas bar-b-que you can imagine, served with a big side of beans cooked with lard, and a big gob of mayonnaise-y potato salad. My grandmother arrived a few hours later to start working on the "blue plate special" of the day – usually some combination of fried chicken, chicken fried steak, meat loaf and gravy, or some equally devilish protein served with mashed potatoes or mac and cheese, and some vegetable that had been boiled to within an inch of its life with copious amounts of bacon fat. Food, the southern, home-cooked kind, was always available, as well as an infinite supply of pre-packaged sweets and soda pop.

Why was I living with my grandparents? Interesting story – I'll tell you the short version, which is about the only version I know.

My mother left my father while she was pregnant with me, and then abandoned me to my grandparents sometime within my first five years of my life (she came and went for the first few years so I'm not exactly sure when it was that she "officially disappeared"). She was a singer who toured with various big bands. I was told she left for a U.S.O. tour and did not return; I found out later that she left with her boyfriend who had gone A.W.O.L. from the service, they abandoned a borrowed car somewhere in Chicago, and the two were never heard from again. And since my grandparents never talked about it, any other history died with them. That's about as much as I know, or will ever know about it, since any other details departed with my grandparents' passing.

My grandparents operated our small café at a bare profit, if any. They were both terrific southern-style home cooks but not terrific business people. They worked hard during the day to make a living, and drank heavily during the evening for lack of one.

It was not exactly *Father Knows Best* around my house. I was often threatened to be taken to an orphanage. And I secretly wished that I would be dropped off at the orphanage, where I was sure some nice, normal couple just like Rob and Laura Petrie from the Dick Van Dyke Show would come along and rescue me. But of course if I had said this, I would have been "switched" within an inch of my life. (Switching, if you don't know, is kind of a southern thing. You take the skinniest little branch you can find from a tree, strip off any leaves which might possibly cushion the blow, and then "switch" it back and forth across the back of the legs. Stings like the dickens. Folks, don't try this at home.)

By my early teens, I was chubby, pimple-y and insecure. Go figure.

At 16, I married my high school sweetheart, mainly as a means of getting out of my house (yeah, that always works out). That lasted about 3 years. My poor, unsuspecting 19-year-old husband had no idea that he was my vehicle to an imagined life. A little unfair, in retrospect.

The Hungry Years

Growing up, I lived vicariously through television. *Leave it to Beaver, I Love Lucy, Ozzie and Harriet* – to me this was everyone else's life besides mine. I memorized things that would be sophisticated to order – café au lait, chateaubriand – so I would know what to order when I started my "real" life. Yes sir, at six years old I was all prepared to order my first dry martini (whatever *that* was).

Once I was "on my own" and determined to live life like the characters I had admired, what followed was a series of just about every diet known to man. I bought every diet book that hit the charts. High this, low that, all of these and none of those. When I was "dieting", I resentfully restrained myself while I sat watching friends enjoy delicious food, and when I wasn't dieting I often over-indulged, partly due to a recent or planned future deprivation.

I maintained a more-or-less acceptable body weight over the years, sometimes a little overweight, sometimes not, through this cycle of yo-yo dieting. But I was never comfortable with how I was eating, and suffered constant feelings of either deprivation or guilt.

The one good thing I got out of all those diets and nutrition books was a pretty good education on the effects of different macronutrients and micronutrients on the body, and what it takes to keep a body running well. What I didn't get was any sort of sustainable plan that didn't involve an obsession with food, measuring something, counting something, or eliminating whole categories of things.

The Road that Led to France

In 2010, my life changed abruptly. My husband (not the 19-year-old one – the one I married 10 years later who was my partner-in-everything and best friend for 28 years), passed away suddenly and unexpectedly. It was a loss more devastating than anything I could have imagined, and one that I don't think I would have survived without my children and dearest friends.

Everyone handles loss differently and gets through it the best they can. A friend of mine confessed to going to Baskin-Robbins and buying one of those enormous tubs of ice cream that they keep in the freezer case, to sustain herself over the course of a week. I even read a story of one woman who ordered a wedding cake and brought the whole thing home for herself, which she devoured over the course of the next few days.

For me it was the opposite. After so many years of cooking meals for my family, I really kind of lost interest in food. Besides, who ever heard of a cookbook called "Cooking for One"?

While the circumstances are those which I would not wish on anyone, it served as sort of a reboot where food is concerned. I didn't really cook anymore and was eating very simply if at all – an egg and a slice of toast, a little sliced turkey and some raw vegetables (why bother cooking them). And to preserve my sanity, I walked. A lot.

Ok, here's where the story gets good again

Time went by and I began to adjust to my new life. Then one day out of the blue, a friend whom I had casually known and admired for over 20 years reached out to me (on Facebook of all things – thanks, Mark Zuckerberg). I found out that he too had lost his wife shortly after my husband passed away. We arranged to get together the next weekend.

That "first date" was pretty magical, and given that we'd known each other for such a long time, we honestly knew from that first night that we would be "a couple". After just a few weeks, he told me he needed to go to Paris on business and asked if I wanted to come with him.

Little did he know, that question was basically like asking someone in hell if they'd care for a glass of ice water.

My first lessons in eating Frenchly

Paris was a place I had always wanted to go, and it was everything I had hoped it would be. The moment I stepped off the plane, I was home.

Beauty was everywhere – the buildings, the people, and of course, the food.

We didn't have much time, only a few days since it was a business trip, but that didn't matter. It was April in Paris. Every moment was fascinating and every restaurant was a new experience. We ate whatever we wanted, whenever we wanted.

And we walked like crazy. From one end of Paris to the other. Why on earth would I want to sit in a taxi when I could stroll down beautiful streets of architectural wonder, stop into cafes for a glass of champagne or freshly made croissant, walk along the river and hear the sounds of street musicians?

Since that first trip to Paris, I've been eating like a French woman; not just the food (which I do enjoy whenever possible) but the whole attitude and approach to food. And I've maintained a consistent weight which, before these changes, I only occasionally and temporarily dipped down to with great struggle and hard work.

We go back to Paris every year, and I confess, on my most recent trips to France, with writing this book in mind, I was a bit of a *voyeur*. When I saw someone who was overweight, I hovered nearby to listen to them speak. Not eavesdropping *per se,* since I wasn't particularly listening to what they were saying (and couldn't understand it anyway). I was only listening to discern whether they were French, or from the U.S. or other parts of the world. And yes, in my very unscientific survey, 100% of the overweight people I observed were speaking English, Spanish, German, and a host of other unrecognizable languages – never French. (I'm sure there must be a few chubby ones somewhere, but maybe they don't go outdoors until they've dropped a few pounds.)

I have found the principles necessary to create a French metabolism, and you don't even have to go to France to have it. But, by all means, go to France whenever you can!

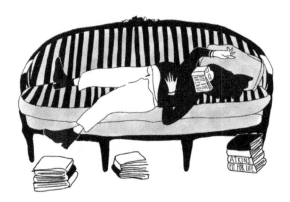

CHAPTER 3
FACT VS. ... *FACT?* THE PROBLEM WITH
DIETS

This is the God's-honest truth – pretty much all diets work, while you're on them. And I should know, I've done most of them. The problem with diets is this – your body is always going to reflect the way you are eating *right now*. And most diets are just not *sustainable* as a way of life.

Here's a little timeline of the things we Americans have done trying to achieve and maintain an ideal weight:

1960's -

Dr. Atkins released his Diet Revolution and the world was taken by storm with this original ketogenic diet. The general idea of this is that you put your body in a state of ketosis by restricting glucose, the preferred fuel of most cells, causing you to burn fat through the release of ketones in the body.

Yes, the diet will cause you to lose weight (remember I said pretty much all diets work) and is a somewhat decent framework for a diet. But there are a few problems:

- Because of the very restricted (20 grams per day) carbohydrate consumption, people tend to eat excessive protein, which can be very hard on the kidneys, plus a lot of poor-quality fats.

- You have to count the carbs (including those in vegetables), and pee on a stick to see if you got it right (the ketosis part). *Some* of us (present company included) would pretty much skip the carbs altogether so we didn't have to count them or pee on the stick, and it just became a good excuse to eat a lot of bacon.

- There are also health concerns over keeping your body in a highly acidic state for any extended period of time.

1970's –

We were big on liquid diets, including Slim Fast and The Last Chance Diet, which did in fact turn out to be a lot of people's last chance. The "Prolinn" drink, a protein drink named after creator Dr. Robert Linn, was made from slaughterhouse leftovers and was taken off the market after the death of some of its consumers.

1980's –

Harvey and Marilyn Diamond released their "Fit for Life" diet and everyone was food combining – fats with carbs or fats with protein, but no mixing of carbs with protein; fruit with nothing but … fruit. The premise was that mis-combining foods would cause them to decompose in your stomach (isn't that what digestion is?) It was a tough diet to stick with, plus you could never eat a hamburger on a bun.

Meal plan programs like Jenny Craig and Nutriystem also gained a lot of popularity in the 80's. These programs are based purely on the "calories in/calories out" theory. It sounds reasonable, but your body doesn't do math quite that way. Different foods affect our bodies in different ways, and go through different metabolic paths, so a calorie doesn't necessarily equal a calorie.

I think these "systems" are the worst possible way to approach weight loss, for a couple of reasons. First, the food (other than a little side salad you may add here or there), being entirely prepared and packaged in advance, is highly processed (more on that later). Second and more importantly, it in no way changes your attitude and approach to eating.

Friends I've seen on these plans have lost weight while they were on them, only to gain all of the weight back, plus more, when they returned to normal eating. I tried one of these programs a number of years ago (I told you I've done them all). I lasted about a week. I was hungry all the time, the food was barely mediocre, and at the end of the first (and only) week I'd gained weight from eating processed foods. Buh-bye.

1990's –

The 90's brought us Susan Powter's "Stop the Insanity" and people were jumping on the non-fat bandwagon. I can't even begin to cover the insanity that diet brought about. You could eat a bag of bagels, but cream cheese? Fuhgettaboudit. Suddenly in stores you saw non-fat versions of everything.

But to make a food that inherently has fat, into a non-fat food, requires massive processing. More sugar, as well as a host of unidentifiable chemicals, must be added to make up for the flavor that is extracted when you remove fat. And the natural composition of the food in terms of nutrients is lost.

2000's –

Early in the 21st century, we were encouraged to become Neanderthals with the paleo diet. The life span of a cave man was about 30 or 40 years. Enough said.

Looking at diet differently

All of these diets can rightfully claim results in weight loss *while on the diet,* but 95% of the people who diet gain the weight back within the first months or years, with many gaining more than was lost.

Meanwhile through all of those decades, the French were enjoying their normal diet of real food composed of the basic macronutrients - protein, carbohydrates and fats, and staying slim in the process. They weren't eliminating the wondrous crusty-on-the-outside-chewy-on-the-inside baguette, they weren't shunning duck l'orange because it combined protein with fruit, and they weren't eating fat free butter.

All of this may make you think, "What's the point of dieting if I'm just going to gain it all back again?" And guess what? You're right! Just to prove a point, nobody can tell you more about diets and what you "should" and "shouldn't" eat than an overweight person, right?

One-third of Americans are on a diet right now, and two-thirds of those people will gain back more weight than they lose. While on a diet, the foods you eat may change, temporarily, but the attitude hasn't.

Dieting is pointless, unless you change your eating way of life.

The primary definition of the word diet is:

1. the kinds of food that a person, animal, or community habitually eats: "a vegetarian diet" synonyms: selection of food, food, foodstuffs, grub, nosh (Oxford Dictionary)

When we think of diet, however, we generally think of the second definition, which is:

2. a special course of food to which one restricts oneself, either to lose weight or for medical reasons: "I'm going on a diet" (Oxford Dictionary)

So what would the ideal diet, or eating way of life be? It would be

- Sustainable, something you can live with from here on out that would maintain your body at a healthy weight without having to completely shun foods that appear at parties or fine restaurants, and that you love.

- Enjoyable, since eating is so much more than just putting nourishment in your body. Eating is celebratory, festive. It brings about a sense of community. When I cook dinner for my family or friends, it isn't because I want to spend more time in the kitchen. It's because I want to bring people together, to nourish mind, body and soul with lingering conversation over caringly prepared food.

- Healthy, because you want to look and feel great for a long time. As Hippocrates said, "Let food be thy medicine and medicine be thy food." Except he said it in Greek.

The French way of eating encompasses all of these elements. It's completely sustainable, because there's nothing you are swearing off of for the rest of eternity, or even for next week necessarily. It's completely enjoyable because you're having real, delicious food, and it's completely healthy because the food you will be eating is fresh and natural.

Even if you do want to follow a specific or more restricted diet (like paleo, vegetarian, vegan), applying the principles in this book will help you reach your goals faster and maintain your weight more easily.

Man was intended to be an omnivorous creature (you can tell by the teeth – we have both the square ones and the pointy ones). Unless you're following a vegan or vegetarian diet for spiritual, medical, or personal reasons, you should be able to enjoy everything that comes under the heading of "food", in its natural form, and in proper proportion.

What is a metabolism, and why do I want a French one?

Metabolism is the physical and chemical processes by which an organism's material substance is produced, maintained and destroyed. The word comes from the Greek *metabol*, change, and *ism*, to throw.

And we're about to throw down some change.

Simplified, it's the chemical reactions that sustain life – the conversion of food to energy, the conversion of that fuel to building blocks of the cells (proteins, lipids and carbohydrates), and the elimination of waste products.

Much has been written and speculated about the "French Paradox" – the fact that France is one of the top five countries with the lowest incidence of heart disease, while consuming a diet high in saturated fat such as cheese and butter.

More to our subject, the French are not normally overweight despite a lifestyle that does not seem conducive to being slender, at least not to the American way of thinking. Croissant, bread, foie gras, butter, and cheese are staples in the French diet. While we're fighting the battle of the bulge in the good ole' US of A, the French are enjoying beautiful, rich sauces such as hollandaise and béarnaise, which sit atop meats and eggs with luscious, runny yolks. Wine is enjoyed, in moderation, often on a daily basis.

How is it that the French just do not get fat?

There are three main factors to firing up your French metabolism which I will be teaching you.

I will also be giving you some key guidelines to incorporate into your life. I would call them "rules", but the French woman would probably rather give birth to a flaming porcupine than follow rules, and besides, this is more about breaking the rules. Still, in learning anything new, it's good to separate out the really important points, so I've summed these up in the end.

As I've said, they are simple – so simple that you may be tempted to blow by them to get to the "meaty parts".

Friends, listen, these *are* the meaty parts.

Whether you follow an omnivore, carnivore, vegetarian or vegan way of eating, the factors and guidelines still apply. This is not so much about specifically *what* you eat as it is about *how* you eat.

You're about to create a whole new lifestyle, a new attitude, and a new way of looking at yourself and at food. So don't be in such an all-fired rush, and commit to each guideline and each change fully.

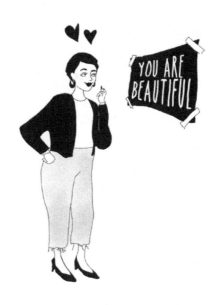

CHAPTER 4
A FRENCH FRAME OF MIND

Before we launch into the three factors you'll be applying to achieve your ideal body, there is one preliminary step to apply, and that is fixing your own mindset.

A mindset is a set of beliefs one has about oneself and one's own qualities and abilities. It is entirely created by you, and entirely changeable by you. And it's more powerful than anything you'll eat.

French Metabolism Guideline – Create a Positive Self-Image, and Wear it with Confidence

To create a French metabolism, you have to shift your mindset.

This is the foundation for change.

The French woman is self-possessed; she is not self-obsessed.

She does not criticize every perceived imperfection, but rather enjoys her own unique qualities.

She enjoys the pleasures of life, and makes adjustments where needed.

What are you telling yourself about *you* every day? That you're a beautiful, sensual creature? That you're taking positive steps and getting better and closer to your goals every day?

Do you shroud yourself in the vision of how you want to look, how you want to feel, and the impression you make on others?

Or are you reminding yourself constantly of your own imagined shortcomings, any past failures, barriers you think you have, and a negative image of yourself?

This mindset is important for two reasons –

First, and listen up, this is a big one – passion is the key to discipline.

Willpower could pretty well be summed up as forcing, or willing, yourself, to do something you don't really want to do or aren't inclined to do. Would you agree?

Alright, so let me ask you – did you ever have to use willpower to do something you're passionate about? I didn't think so.

Willpower leads to frustration. Passion leads to motivation.

You can fire up your passion just by having a good look at what you want to achieve, or what you want to avoid. Then feed that passion daily with your vision of yourself.

Since you're reading this book, I'm going to go out on a limb here and assume that you are someone who wants to achieve and maintain your idea of an ideal weight. That you would like to put on fashionable clothes and have them look the way you'd like to see yourself. That you'd like to climb stairs or take a hike without carrying the equivalent of a 10 or 20 or 30 pound box around with you all the time.

To start getting your passion fired up, ask yourself some clarifying questions –

How will achieving my ideal weight make me feel physically? Do I want to be more active? More agile? Less tired?

How will it affect my overall attitude and confidence? Do I want to be less self-conscious about my appearance?

How will I be able to dress at my new weight? Are there clothes I would love to wear, that I just can't wear at my current weight?

What will happen if I don't change what I'm currently doing? Is my current way of eating leading me to an unhealthy future?

Take the time to clearly identify these for yourself, to fuel your commitment in the choices you make.

Second, your decisions about yourself are powerful things. You must take the time to visualize what you want to look like, so your body knows where it's going. After all, how can you achieve a goal you haven't set?

It may sound cliché but it's true, if you can't see it, you can't be it. You have to tell your body what it's supposed to do.

This is an important exercise that I want you to fully devote yourself to.

Choose a calm, quiet time when you're not distracted with work or kids or television – maybe while you're still lying in bed in the morning before the chaos of the world has started, or at the end of the day while you're drifting off to sleep.

Get a good, clear picture in your mind of what you intend to look like. What's your overall size? What do your arms look like? What do your legs look like? What about your tummy and butt? How do you want to dress and present yourself? Be as detailed as possible.

But here's the tricky part, it has to be *you* – your height, your age, your realistically ideal body. Not Penelope Cruz' head on top of Beyonce's body, or any other wild combination. Don't picture yourself as 5'11 if you're 5'2 (fun-size, like me). Or as a 25-year-old if you're 50.

It may take a few minutes, a few hours, or even a few tries, but keep at it and don't give up. Eventually you'll come up with an image that is you, at your age, your height, and your optimum body.

Don't freak out, I'm not getting all metaphysical on you. We're just setting the stage, putting the goal there, and starting right here and right now to live the life you're going to live from here on out.

Start walking around with a positive self-image right now, with what you've got and where you're at right now. Look at it in your quiet time regularly, and remind yourself that you're getting closer every day.

Just that little shift in how you think about yourself can be life-changing. But don't worry, we're not stopping there. Not by a long shot.

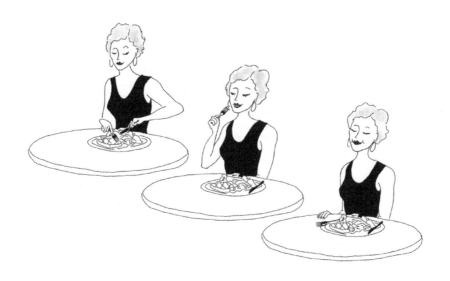

CHAPTER 5
THE FIRST FACTOR – YOUR
RELATIONSHIP WITH FOOD

Here it is, the first big factor in creating a French Metabolism – your relationship with the food you eat. And by *relationship*, I mean your general attitude and connection with food.

Let me tell you right up front that, like the French, I love food. I look forward to great meals with complete anticipation, and search out Michelin-starred restaurants like a dog hunts a bone. I've never been one of those people who are ambivalent about food or forget to eat. In fact, it's one of my great passions in life along with family, friends, and France.

Americans have unfortunately confused quantity with quality. Many popular diets are based on the premise that you can eat *unlimited quantities* of *this*, as long as you never eat *that*. These diets are not only generally unhealthy, they enable the problem by feeding into the notion that an excessive quantity of food is acceptable or even desirable. And while they may be workable on a short term basis, you will need to resolve not to eat *that* for the rest of your life in order to maintain your weight loss.

The truth is, you just don't need to eat *unlimited quantities* of anything.

A French attitude toward food is much more about quality than quantity. And because you know you can eat anything you want, you don't have to eat everything, all the time, all at once.

Let's get some perspective on quantity. You've probably heard or read before that your stomach is about the size of your fist. Go ahead, look at that balled-up fist right now. That's not exactly true for everyone, but let's agree that the empty stomach is a relatively small organ. That same miraculous little stomach is capable of expanding up to *50 times* its empty volume when a large meal is consumed!

But think about it – your stomach was *full* when you ate that first, fist'ish-sized portion of food!

We'll address why you have the urge to sometimes overeat (and why it's not your fault) very thoroughly in the next factor. But the first change in mindset is that *you don't need to eat a lot of food to feel satisfied.*

One fairly consistent difference between overweight and slender people is this: overweight people tend to attack their food, whereas slender people eat slowly, like a cat playing with a mouse. Why is this significant?

When you consume food with rapid vigor, you often don't

realize you're full until you've already overeaten. And worse, we can come to be so accustomed to that overly-full feeling when we've eaten, that it begins to feel normal.

Let's talk biology for a minute. I could get all technical and talk about the role of the hypothalamus and blood sugar levels which signal hunger and satiety (the feeling that you've had enough and it's time to quit eating) in the brain.

But since the French woman doesn't get all caught up in the technical details, let's just say that there's a whole lot of complex signaling that tells you when you've had enough to eat, and those signals take longer to tell you you're full, than the amount of time it takes to stretch your stomach to 50 times its original size, if you are eating very fast.

French Metabolism Guideline – Put. The Fork. Down.

Here is an exercise I want you to consciously and deliberately commit to for at least the next couple of weeks. It may be the most important thing in this book, and may be the only thing you will need to do to get your weight under control. I can't overstate how important this is.

For the next two weeks, I want you to commit to very deliberately putting your fork (or spoon or chopsticks or sandwich or whatever) *down* after *each and every bite* you take. Actually take it out of your hand and place it on the plate. It's not enough to just hold onto the fork and pause while you chew and swallow – Put. It. Down. And refuse to pick it up again until you have *completely* chewed your food to a pulp and swallowed the previous bite.

As you'll soon see, this is *a lot* harder than it sounds. We get very accustomed to shoveling up the next bite while still chewing the last one. But honestly, you can only eat one bite of food at a time, right? Also, with that next bite poised on the fork while still chewing the last, we tend to chew less and swallow faster, denying the digestive enzymes their job of breaking down food into nutrient particles that the body can absorb. You don't have teeth in your stomach, you know.

If you have a spouse or partner, get them to help you (if you can get them to do it with you, it will be good for them, too). It will be annoying as hell, but remind each other each time you fail to put down the utensil before the next bite.

Shoveling up the next bite while eating the current one is a tough habit to break, and you'll be shocked to see how automatic this is. When I started adopting this behavior I was catching myself pretty much every other bite, and I've never considered myself a fast eater!

You won't have to deliberately do this bite-after-bite for the rest of your life. But after a couple of weeks of this (or as long as you need to do it) it will become second nature to pause, chew, and enjoy your food before taking another bite.

Continue to do this *consciously* until you have naturally slowed your pattern of eating. When you do this, two things are going to happen.

One, you give those wonderful signaling hormones and nerve receptors time to tell your brain you are full, instead of having to have your overstretched stomach tell you.

The second thing that happens when you slow down and put your fork down between every bite, is that you are going to be amazed to discover what a small amount of food is actually required for you to feel satisfied and "full".

Which leads to our next point.

French Metabolism Guideline – Don't Eat if you're not Hungry,

and when you're Full, Stop Eating.

You may feel full so quickly in fact, that you worry you haven't eaten enough to "last" until the next meal. Well, just remember that fist-sized stomach. And besides, guess what the body runs on when it runs out of quickly available energy? Fat reserves! Isn't that what we want?

Your body is pretty smart, it will tell you when it needs food (as you well know). There's absolutely no benefit to forcing yourself to eat, or to continue to eat when you aren't hungry.

It's obvious that, on the one hand, eating too much food (in excess of what we need) causes weight gain. On the other hand, eating too little food (as in extreme dieting) slows the metabolism. It's almost "damned if you do, damned if you don't".

The natural, French solution to this are the two guidelines above, eating slowly enough that the body registers fullness through metabolic signaling, not an overly-full stomach, and stopping when you are no longer hungry.

French Metabolism Guideline – It's Okay to Feel a Little Hungry Between Meals

Unless you're super-thin or undernourished (in which case you probably wouldn't be reading this), feeling hungry doesn't mean you're going to starve.

Hunger (unless you are literally starving – and by literally, I mean *literally*) is simply a sensation, it's not a B-52 crater. It is the result of a shift in various hormone levels, which we'll look at very shortly.

Later on, I have some quick and easy suggestions for how to deal with hunger between meals.

> *French Metabolism Guideline – Eat all you* **Need** *to eat, not all you* **Can** *eat.*

Super-size and all-you-can-eat are really an American thing, again confusing quantity with quality.

Even at all-you-can-eat salad bars, I've watched overweight people pile their oversized plate with gloppy, mayonnaise-y dishes that are anything but salad, and anything but healthy.

An interesting little story, I was traveling in Europe with a group of Americans, and the restaurant where we ate one evening offered a salad bar for the first course. One member of our group piled his plate with salad, typical of American salad bar eaters. When the bill arrived, he was charged for two salad bars, since, from the European perspective, "no single person eats that much!"

You've probably heard the phrase, "Eat like a king at breakfast, a prince at lunch and a pauper at dinner." In France, the phrase would be more like this: "Eat every meal like a king in quality and a pauper in quantity." When you choose wholesome food, which we will look at in detail later, and you take the time to eat slowly and recognize when you are satisfied, you realize you don't need a large volume of food.

If you're one of those people who thinks that if they go to a buffet, they must keep eating to "get their money's worth", then don't go to buffets, at least not until you've adjusted your relationship with food. Or learn to accept the fact that whatever you paid is the price for a satisfying meal, regardless of the size, and quit when you are satisfied. It's a bigger waste to consume food you don't need, than to spend a little extra money on a smaller meal.

> *French Metabolism Guideline – Eat at Meal Times, and Don't Skip Meals.*

Skipping meals as a solution to weight loss usually backfires. It results in getting too hungry, followed by eating too much, too fast.

The French way of eating includes eating moderate meals three times a day, at meal times. In fact, aside from Paris which is more tourist-oriented, most restaurants are not even open outside of normal meal times.

The French do not snack or eat "mini-meals" throughout the day, which research shows creates a constant circulation of insulin, a fat-promoting hormone, in the body. It also tends to keep your attention on food throughout the day, and sometimes those mini-meals aren't so mini.

When you eat sufficient food at mealtimes, you have time to focus on and enjoy the foods you are eating.

It's true that going too long without eating can slow the metabolism, but "too long" is more like 6 or 7 hours, not 2 or 3. The only exception to "no snacking" might be a light nibble in the late afternoon, since the French tend to eat dinner quite late. But this would be a few nuts or olives or a piece of fruit, or maybe a little bread and cheese.

French Metabolism Guideline – Drink Plenty of Water

There is one thing the French do fill up on throughout the day, and that's water. Not only does water fill the stomach, giving a temporary feeling of satiety, it also promotes beautiful skin and proper elimination (when you "lose" weight, how do you think it leaves the body? Elimination!)

There's so many things water does for us, I could write a book just on that subject. It helps give you a clear, moist complexion, removes waist and unwanted fat from the body, and allows blood to pump more freely through the body, just to name a few.

My husband was a reluctant water-drinker, only willing to drink it if it were flavored with something or a certain temperature, until I made the comparison that drinking water is like going to the bathroom – you don't go because you want to, you don't go only if the seat is warm and fuzzy. No, you go because you need to. Same with drinking water.

Another bonus, if you're feeling a little hungry between meals, drinking a couple glasses of water will give you that sensation of fullness that will probably be sufficient to hold you over to the next meal. I know, *"Yum, I'll have a big glass of water,"* said no one ever. But it works.

In case you're worried about water intoxication (hyponatremia), don't. This is a condition that results from drinking an extreme amount of water in a short amount of time, which dilutes the salt levels in the blood. It's a very serious condition, and can be fatal.

How much would you have to drink for that to occur? Literally gallons and gallons. This mainly occurs in athletes who grossly overestimate their need for water replacement. In the normal course of a day this is just not going to happen, even if you're sipping water all day long.

How much water should you be drinking? It's different for everyone, because we all come in different sizes and do different activities. But a good rule of thumb is – half your body weight, in ounces. In other words, a 120 pound human should be drinking about 60 ounces of water a day, or about a gallon.

Meeting your "quota" may take a bit of concerted effort until you get used to it. Consider filling a gallon jug each morning, or using a one-quart water bottle (which you'll fill up four times), or some other method of making sure you get enough water. I believe you'll be very pleasantly surprised with just this change alone.

French Metabolism Guideline – After Dinner, the Kitchen is Closed

As I've said earlier, the French do not snack, and that includes after dinner. When dinner is done, eating is done.

Dinner should be adequately satisfying, and may even include a glass of wine and a small sweet or piece of fruit. You should feel sufficiently full, and in just a few hours you'll go to sleep and your hunger hormones will shift, as we'll talk about shortly.

I think one of the best deterrents to night-time nibbling is cleaning the kitchen. It puts a big "Sorry, we're closed" sign on the kitchen and an exclamation point on the fact that eating is done.

If you just have to have that late night treat, enjoy a cup of chamomile or other herbal tea.

French Metabolism Guideline – Monitor, and Moderate

When I see someone who is quite overweight, I know that, at some point, they just stopped paying attention.

We monitor the things we are concerned with and want to be in control of. A business person continually monitors sales and profits to ensure their actions are resulting in growth. An active stock market investor is monitoring movement of stocks to make quick changes that protect and increase their investment. If your child is running a fever, you check it repeatedly to make sure it's going down, and take action if it isn't. And if you want to create and maintain an ideal body size, you have to know where you stand, what is bringing you closer to the goal, and what creates set-backs.

French women generally monitor their weight with their hands – how their body feels or how their clothes fit. But for me, this means stepping on the scale every morning – it's just part of my morning rituals like brushing my teeth. I want to be on top of small fluctuations in my weight so I can moderate as needed.

Whether judging by the number on the scale or the fit of favorite jeans, the French woman monitors and innately moderates her eating to control her weight. What does that look like in action? Simply put, it's just balancing things out.

You will never hear a French woman bemoaning, "my God, all the *calories*!" or "I shouldn't have eaten that!" If she wants to enjoy an indulgence, she does, in moderation (since it is not part of the mindset to eat vast quantities), and then compensates for it as needed.

If you've gone to a party or special dinner the night before, spend the next day (or two or three or whatever it takes) enjoying fruits and vegetables, salads and broth-based soups. Get in some extra activity. Balance things out quickly and don't let unwanted pounds add up.

Even better, if you know you'll be attending a function where a big meal will be served, plan to eat conservatively a few days in advance. But don't use this as an excuse to go "hog wild", just enjoy your meal in your new, regular manner, pausing between bites and stopping when you're full, and it will all come out just fine.

French Metabolism Guideline – Get Enough Sleep

Have you ever noticed that when you don't get enough sleep, you're hungry all day? Well, it's not all in your head – there's a real reason for that.

Let me introduce you to two hormones, leptin (the hormone that makes you feel satisfied), and ghrelin (the hormone that signals hunger).

Here's what happens – when you sleep, leptin increases, allowing you to go seven or eight hours without waking up in the middle of the night from hunger. At the same time, ghrelin decreases, so that it's not sending you signals that you need to wake up and eat. Think of it as if they're riding a teeter-totter. (Thanks, hormones.)

When you don't get adequate sleep, the result is a decrease in leptin and an excess of ghrelin in your system, sending signals to you all day telling you that you are hungry. Ahhhh, that explains it!

Picture a French film, the femme fatale lying languidly between cool sheets, deliciously enjoying her sleep. More than just a sexy image, she's restoring her body, improving her appearance, and balancing her hunger-craving hormones.

I've never been someone who just loves sleep (how many times did I used to say "I'll sleep when I'm dead"), so I've had to work on sleeping like a French woman. I've made my bed an oasis that keeps me swaddled and tempted to stay for that extra hour or two. I've switched to Belgian linen sheets which have an amazing organic texture, added a memory foam topper that swallows me up with coziness, and a soft, down comforter. And I top it all off with diffusing lavender oil in the room. Yep, it's pretty great.

Do what you need to do that keeps you comfortably between the sheets for the seven or eight hours, or whatever you need, to be fully rested, and keep the ghrelin gremlin from dominating the see-saw.

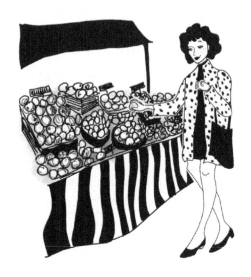

CHAPTER 6
THE SECOND FACTOR – THE QUALITY OF FOOD YOU EAT

Here's that next big factor, so pay attention. One of the biggest culprits that could be sabotaging your weight is the inherent quality of the food you are eating.

Engineered Foods

What if I told you it's not your fault? That you, my American friend, have been engineered to fail?

It's true, we have been duped. Played. Bamboozled. American processed foods and fast foods have been engineered with chemicals to make us crave more and eat more, using components otherwise used to make yoga mats and antifreeze.

If you live in the United States, you have been eating genetically engineered foods since the 1990's, with approximately 60% of all processed foods on supermarket shelves containing engineered ingredients.

To make matters worse, processed foods are engineered to stimulate dopamine, that feel-good neurotransmitter causing food cravings and addiction.

Conversely, in France and other European countries, GMOs and pesticides have been banned, and most foods are minimally processed.

GMO research began in the early 1900's, with the goal of creating food that would be cheaper, more plentiful, and have a longer shelf-life. What this means for the manufacturer is increased time to get products to the market, longer shelf-life and greater profits. What that means for you and me is chemical and biological sabotage.

I am not a scientist and am not qualified to give a full dissertation on the dangers of chemical additives and GMOs – truthfully I don't think even the scientists know fully the dangers of GMOs and certain additives.

However, I don't need to be a scientist to state with certainty that the human body is designed to use real food for fuel, breaking it down into nutrients that can nourish the various organs, and maintain the balance that makes a healthy body.

When you introduce fake, engineered, non-foods into the diet, the body does not innately know what to do with these. So, apparently, it shoves it someplace while it tries to figure it out. The result? More you. Not in a good way.

Then there's preservatives. Preservatives are things that can't be consumed by bacteria. But how does digestion occur? Bacteria! That friendly gut bacteria, lactobacillus, helps to break down food so it can be digested and absorbed, and used to nourish the body.

That big box store jumbo sized, 24 count pack of anything that can sit on your shelf for the next three to forty years? Poor lactobacillus doesn't stand a chance at breaking that down.

Why is it that people can eat bread in Europe and not gain weight, but eating bread in America blows you up like the Michelin man?

In France, the baker is up pre-dawn, making bread from wheat that grows high in the field, which will be purchased that day and consumed in the next day or two. It's made to slowly rise and naturally ferment, so it's easy to digest.

In America, typical bread is factory made in the quickest way possible, and engineered to hold up to transporting on a truck, where it is then on the grocery shelf for a few days before some poor, unsuspecting soul picks it up. Most breads in America are made from dwarf wheat, which was developed through cross-breeding and genetic modification around the 1960's, and is prepared using quick-rise yeast which short-cuts the process of sprouting and fermenting, important for digestion.

That explains a lot, right? Yes, I know there are those who are gluten intolerant (about 1% of the population), but I believe most people are "additive intolerant", "preservative intolerant", or "GMO intolerant".

That's the bad news. The good news is we know the culprit and can do something about it.

French Metabolism Guideline – Avoid Highly Processed Foods

You hear a lot about processed foods, but what does that mean exactly?

Essentially, processed foods are any foods that have been altered prior to consumption.

A couple of years ago, I had the occasion to live in Hungary for a couple of months (long story, different book). I rented an apartment rather than opting to stay in a hotel, so I could sort of "live" there, settle in, and cook my own meals.

One thing I was utterly unprepared for was the grocery stores – everything was in Hungarian. I know, duh, right? I had traveled to countries like France and Spain where, while the words were foreign, there was still similarity because many of our words are European in origin. But Hungarian is a language fully unto itself, and I couldn't make out a word of it.

I subsisted on only whole, real ingredients that I could recognize – fresh fruits and vegetables (which are only available seasonally, by the way), eggs, cheeses, and of course my nose led me to regular stops at the fresh bakery.

I did venture to buy a can of tuna once, thinking I could add it to a salad, but when I opened it I wasn't sure if it was for human or cat consumption so, lacking a cat, I tossed it out.

The result of this was that I lost about 8 pounds without even attempting to lose weight. I had great energy, and my skin was bright and clear.

It's very unlikely that you are going to make your own yogurt from the fresh milk you took from your cow this morning, or preserve your own fresh vegetables, or flash-freeze your freshly picked blueberries at the peak of ripeness. But what you *can* do is buy as many fresh, seasonal, natural ingredients as possible and choose good quality, organic items when you must buy "lightly" processed foods.

French Metabolism Guideline – Eat at Home

While we think of French food as elaborate dishes with complex sauces (and they certainly can be), and meals that go on for hours (which they certainly can), most meals are simple and homemade.

A study done by the French Commission on Health Education revealed that 75% of people in France eat lunch and dinner at home. Food is purchased from the local market, butcher, baker every few days and consumed fresh. Fast food is no part of the French lifestyle.

Like the French, I love going out to a nice restaurant for a special meal. But, like the French, the majority of my meals are simple, and prepared at home. Restaurant portions, especially in America, tend to be hugely oversized and prepared with ingredients that don't need to be eaten on a regular basis.

Going to a restaurant is a special occasion, where you indulge as you please on reasonable-sized portions, and then return to moderate, simple eating.

You can prepare simple, delicious meals at home in less time than it takes to eat out or have food delivered from a restaurant. And with the loads of money you'll save, you'll have the resources to buy new clothes for your slender, new body.

On our most recent trip to France, we had the privilege of being invited to have lunch with friends in their home just outside of Paris. The meal was simple and amazing. It started with oysters on the half shell, purchased fresh from the local fish shop. This was followed by beouf bourguignon fondue and a mix of roasted green beans, mushrooms and potatoes. The beef was lean and delicious, and it really slows the meal down when you are cooking one bite at a time, plus it's just fun.

After the main meal, an assortment of cheeses and a light salad were served, followed by a fruit crumble prepared from fresh apples and berries picked from the garden, with a shortbread topping. All of this was simple, required minimal preparation, and was one of the best meals we had on our vacation.

Here in America, we don't normally have the advantage of having a fresh baker, butcher or produce market just around the corner. However, most cities these days have Farmer's Markets, as well as grocery stores featuring natural and organic foods.

Later I'll give you more examples of simple meals you can prepare at home or even make ahead, along with a list of kitchen staples and easy, delicious recipes.

French Metabolism Guideline – Buy the Best Food you Can

Buying fresh, organic ingredients used to mean spending a small fortune at a "health-food" store. Today, thanks largely to consumer demand, organic options are popping up in virtually every store. But be aware – you do need to look for the "Certified Organic" symbol to be sure it is organic; words like "wholesome" and "natural" are completely unregulated and may mean nothing except that they cost more.

If you aren't able to buy everything organic, then at least avoid buying the "dirty dozen" – the fruits and vegetables found to have the most residual pesticides – in anything other than organic form. The current dirty dozen list includes:

1. Strawberries
2. Spinach
3. Nectarines
4. Apples
5. Peaches
6. Pears

7. Cherries
8. Grapes
9. Celery
10. Tomatoes
11. Sweet Bell Peppers
12. Potatoes

When it comes to meat, fish and poultry, fresh-caught or well sourced and hormone free can get quite expensive, but it's best to prefer quality over quantity, so consider smaller portions and buy the best you can. Likewise eggs (which by the way are not a breakfast protein in France but are more typically served at lunch or dinner) should be GMO and hormone free.

One more thing for you to know – almost all of the corn and corn products in America are genetically modified unless you buy organic. Likewise, if a product lists "sugar" in the ingredients instead of "cane sugar", it is very likely beet sugar, and, like corn, most of the beets grown in America are genetically modified.

French Metabolism Guideline – Buy Local and Seasonal

While the thought of eating strawberries in the winter or pomegranate in the summer may be appealing, it just isn't natural. Fruits and vegetables made available out of season are often raised in other countries where they must be picked before they have ripened, and treated with gasses and other agents to preserve them so they make it to the store. The result is added chemicals and not much flavor.

Many towns have Farmer's Markets, where local, small farmers sell freshly picked and often organic produce (just ask the vendor if you're not sure).

There are many advantages to purchasing food this way. You know it is fresh (most vendors will let you sample, and you can unmistakably taste the difference). You are supporting local farming. You get to stroll around in the fresh air and chat with other people (very French). And oddly, when I purchase fresh food from the people who have been involved in raising it, I feel like I've sort of "adopted" their food. I'm more likely to lovingly prepare and enjoy it, and less likely to leave it in that drawer in the fridge that you may have thought up to now was specially devised for rotting vegetables.

French Metabolism Guideline – Don't Bother Eating Food that Doesn't Taste Good

Educate your palate to appreciate quality.

We usually think of chefs as having a "refined palate". This is true, but a well-trained palate is learned, it's not something you're necessarily born with.

It isn't difficult to learn. Start by consciously identifying the five main tastes – sweet, sour, bitter, salty, and umami.

What the heck is umami? Okay – geek alert – it's the Japanese word for "yummy" that technically refers to glutamate, an amino acid, with a pleasant, savory flavor. It's a flavor unto itself, not exactly sweet, sour, salty or bitter, and is used to describe such things as mushrooms, meats and some cheeses.

Many foods are a combination of the basic "tastes", for example a lemon tart is both sweet and sour; cheeses can be both salty and umami. The best dishes are a balance of flavors.

Now that you've slowed down your eating, you can take the time to savor your food and think about what you're tasting. Once you've started identifying the basic tastes, start identifying the individual flavors. Start to pick up different fresh herbs – dill, cilantro, parsley, rosemary, thyme, and spices – cinnamon, nutmeg, cumin, and that "what is it?" flavor that is often cardamom. Taste each of these things in their "pure" form so you become familiar with them.

Now it's time to get a little crazy. Start trying new and exotic things (you may have to make another change of mindset about what you do or don't like). Start adding one new fruit or veggie you've never tried, to your weekly shopping list. Add lamb chops and fresh fish and shellfish to your list of usual proteins.

When you start refining your palate, a couple of things happen –

- You slow down your eating to appreciate what you're tasting, and as a result you become more satisfied with less food.

- You lose your taste for highly processed, mass consumption foods, because they just don't taste good anymore.

French Metabolism Guideline – Eat Your Veggies

If you aren't a fan of veggies, I'd venture to say you're doing it wrong.

Growing up in the south, most people had gardens and we had an abundance of fresh vegetables. But unfortunately, they were mostly prepared by boiling them to an over-cooked mush or frying them to a crispy cinder. And salad? I don't think I even knew there was another lettuce besides iceberg until I was in my 20's, and dressings were all a creamy white goo.

Maybe that's why you find so many "meat-and-potato" eaters in the south.

The French diet includes a rainbow of fresh, seasonal fruits and vegetables prepared in the most delicious ways – roasted, confit, blanched, poached and grilled. These methods are not only much healthier than boiling or frying the bejeezus out of them, they also intensify flavors and add texture.

Make a conscious effort to "eat the rainbow", fruits and vegetables in different colors. The colors of fruits and vegetables are a result of the various nutrients they contain. And while I could go into a long, geeky dissertation on what each color represents, if you just eat them all you get the whole enchilada (but without the enchilada, which doesn't really contain much vegetables).

Try new things like roasting sun chokes, grilling radicchio, or sautéing bok choy. Later I'll give you some recommendations on how to make vegetables a favorite part of your meal. Or the whole meal.

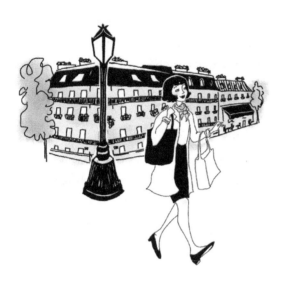

CHAPTER 7
THE THIRD FACTOR – MOVEMENT
(A.K.A. EXERCISE)

When I see weight loss plans promoting that you can "lose weight without exercise", I cringe. It's not that I (or any French woman) am really into hard-core exercise, and it's true that technically you *can* lose weight without exercise. What I object to is the notion that exercise is bad, unpleasant, or something you should want to avoid.

Exercise lowers blood pressure and cholesterol. It increases confidence and libido, and elevates mood. It improves muscle tone and balances energy. And it helps burn up the little "indulgences".

The French woman does not spend hour after hour at the gym. She has no use for hard, masculine muscles. But she exercises aplenty by living an active life and doing the activities of her choosing.

The typical French woman logs thousands of steps per day,

walking through the city or carrying bags of groceries home from the market. She may go to the gym once or twice a week, if she wants to, or may go to a Pilates or yoga class, or ride a bike, or play tennis, or some other activity she enjoys. But she lives an active life and moves often and a lot.

French Metabolism Guideline – Move Every Day

No matter what your fitness level, you can do *something*.

I saw a story a few years ago about a man who, after years of horrible eating and a completely sedentary life, had ballooned to over 500 pounds. He could barely walk himself to the bathroom, and, needless to say, his life was miserable He quite literally sat on his couch all day eating junk food and "trolling" people on the internet.

He finally reached his breaking point and knew he had to change his life.

He started by sitting on the couch making "running" motions *just with his arms* for as long as he could, a few times a day. In a few weeks, his fitness had improved and he was able to pace back and forth from the couch to the kitchen, which he did for as long and as many times a day as possible. A few weeks after that, he was able to start walking outside.

He continued increasing whatever he could do, bit by little bit, as his fitness level and confidence improved, until finally he had achieved a weight loss of over 250 pounds! He still had farther to go to reach his goal (and the show gave him a gift of skin surgery which was necessary for the extreme amount of weight loss). But it just goes to prove that *it is never too late*, and *you can always do something.*

French Metabolism Guideline – Walk Whenever and Wherever you Can

Remember the scene in LA Story, where Steve Martin hops in his car and drives to his neighbor's house?

Here in America we don't really have the mindset of walking to destinations. Cities here tend to be more spread out with less neighborhood spots to visit, so walking is more of a deliberate activity. But it's one of the best exercises you can do for maintaining your weight.

Walking a mile expends about the same amount of energy (about 100 calories) regardless of the speed you are walking. In other words, you can run a mile in about 8 or 10 minutes and you've burned 100 calories in 8 or 10 minutes, or you can walk a mile in 15 minutes and you've burned up about 100 calories in 15 minutes, or you can stroll along the same mile at a 20-25 minute pace and you've burned 100 calories in 20-25 minutes.

The main difference is in cardiovascular fitness – to exercise the heart muscle, one of my favorite muscles, you need to be moving at a clip that gets your heart pumping. Also if you're strolling along at too slow a pace, it's doubtful you'll stay at it the 3 or 4 hours it could take to do some real good.

To be entirely, un-Frenchly technical, here's the deal – to achieve cardiovascular health, you need to be in your aerobic target zone. Your aerobic target zone is around 55 – 85% of your maximum heart rate.

To calculate this, you first need to know your maximum heart rate. This varies for different individuals but a good rough calculation of this is 220 minus your age (for example, if you are 45 years old, 220 – 45 = 175 bpm – beats per minute).

To be exercising aerobically in this example, you'd need to achieve a heart rate of between 55% of 175 (96 bpm) and 85% of 175 (149 bpm). I serious doubt the French bother with calculating all this

– they just walk really fast.

Ideally aim for at least half an hour. Able to do more? Great! Only have 15 or 20 minutes? Do it!

You have a gym the size of the world right outside your door.

French Metabolism Guideline – Stay Active Throughout the Day

There are a billion-jillion ways to incorporate movement into your daily life. For example:

- Do some squats while waiting for the coffee to brew in the morning.

- Curl a dumbbell while talking on the phone (don't forget to switch arms).

- Clean your own house.

- Garden.

- Walk the dog.

- Take the stairs whenever possible.

- Park farther away in the parking lot, or down the street.

- Walk to the coffee shop, dry cleaner or market.

- Have an "active" date with a friend or significant other, like tennis, swimming or playing on the beach.

It's not un-French to do some plain, old-fashioned exercise. You can maintain decent muscle tone spending only 15 or 20 minutes several times a week doing some exercises in addition to your generally active life.

I like to spend a little time every morning after my walk, working upper body, core and legs on alternating days while I watch the news. I'm already in a "movement" frame of mind and can catch up on world events at the same time.

When should you exercise? Hands-down morning is best, for a couple of reasons. First, it's done before the day interferes, as days do, with your best laid plans. Second, it gets the feel-good endorphins going and puts you in a great frame of mind for the day.

But if you just can't do mornings, then "whenever you can" is the best time of day.

Whatever you choose or whenever you do it, just remember the passion principle – make it something you will enjoy or something that will motivate you because of the expected outcome – and stick with it.

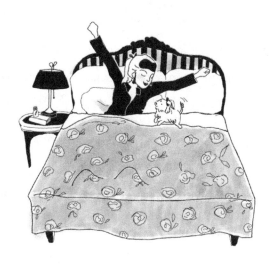

CHAPTER 8
PUTTING IT ALL TOGETHER

Now you have the 3 Factors that create a French metabolism –

Your Relationship With Food

The Quality of Food

Movement

along with your French Metabolism Guidelines. Let's see what creating the French metabolism looks like in action.

You wake up in the morning refreshed after a good night's sleep. There's maybe the faint smell of lavender oil that you applied the night before to relax and get great sleep.

You may start your morning with a cup of coffee or tea, and you'll down a big glass of water or two, which will start to rehydrate you and likely fire up your elimination.

Get in some activity by going for a walk, bike ride, walking the dog, a morning workout, or whatever you enjoy. Then get yourself ready for the day, looking your best for the body type you have right now and feeling positive and confident. You'll notice how your clothes are fitting (or weigh yourself if you prefer) and take note whether you need to adjust your eating for the day or week.

Mid-morning, or whenever you're hungry, you break your long night's fast with a light breakfast, taking a few minutes to sit and enjoy what you're having.

You remain active throughout the day by taking the stairs, parking a distance from your destination, working at a stand-up desk, or moving when possible. And of course sipping water through the day.

Later in the day, around noon or 1:00 (or when you're hungry), you'll have a satisfying, balanced lunch, not too big, not too little (we'll talk about portions in a minute), which you will *sit down* to eat. You take time to chew and enjoy your food, deliberately putting the fork down between bites until you've learned to pace yourself.

If you get a little hungry before dinner, remember it's not the end of the world. But if you need a light snack to get you through the day, you'll have a little handful of nuts or a slice of cheese, or perhaps a piece of seasonal fruit.

At dinner time, you'll prepare your final meal of the day. It will be simple, balanced, delicious, and appropriately sized to keep you satisfied until morning. After dinner, the kitchen is closed.

On a typical day, all of your food will be wholesome and seasonal, and organic whenever possible. You'll avoid fast food or highly processed foods, and in a very short time you will no longer crave any of those things – you'll just have a healthy appetite for delicious, real food.

Eating out in a restaurant is for treats, and no French woman goes to a restaurant to eat a "diet" meal, so enjoy and moderate, and spend the next day or two balancing things out by eating salads and broth-based soups.

Portion size

Bodies are pretty clever things. When you cut yourself, they regenerate skin. When you're tired they send signals that you should rest. When you need to eat, they let you know by way of hunger, and when you're full they tell you when to stop eating. Once you've adjusted the pace and pleasure of how you eat, that's really all you need to know about portions.

However, if you eat very fast, or if you've been eating non-food food, or if you're accustomed to having an overly-full tummy tell you when to stop eating, the signaling may have gotten a little haywire.

The French metabolism guidelines course-corrects this missed signaling, by making you slow down, and by eating real food that nourishes you. But while your body's getting the hang of it, let's take a look at what a normal portion should be.

Proteins

Meat, fish and chicken – usually about 4 – 6 ounces is a decent serving of protein, or, as they say, about the size of a deck of cards or the palm of your hand.

Eggs – 2 eggs are a fairly typical serving. Once you slow down, you may find that one may be enough, especially if it's served with another protein such as bacon or another meat.

Dairy – ½ to 1 cup of yogurt is typically sufficient, or a few slices of cheese.

Vegetables – if they're being served in a somewhat "natural" state, in a salad or soup, sautéed or roasted, you can eat vegetables to your heart's content. They're quite filling so they're really hard to overeat. Creamy, sauce-y preparations are for treats and not part of the daily menu.

Fruits – the French diet typically will include 2 or 3 pieces of fruit a day. It may be added to a recipe or salad, or eaten in its natural state as a snack, or for dessert in the evening.

Breads and grains – since the French do not overeat, these are not excluded from the diet. About a half cup of grains, and a slice or two of bread, or a tartine or croissant, would be eaten in a typical day.

Fats – again, since food is not being over-eaten, these are not restricted. No one is going to eat a stick of butter or drink a cup of oil. A little pat of butter on bread, or salad or vegetables prepared with a tablespoon or two of good oil for flavoring, should be enough to do the trick.

Herbs, spices and seasonings – these are used liberally in preparing delicious, home cooked meals. Fresh herbs are rich in phytochemicals and micronutrients, and give a wonderful burst of fresh flavor. Typically, herbs which grow on soft stems (basil, parsley, dill) can be used in raw form, and those on a more woody stem (rosemary, oregano) are used in cooking.

What about sugar?

French desserts are quite amazing, but sweets are not a regular part of the French diet, and desserts, when eaten, are very small.

When the French indulge in a restaurant meal it would most certainly include dessert, but the portion would normally be less than half the size of most of our portions in America. Otherwise, dessert would be a piece of fruit, some fresh berries, or a square or two of dark chocolate.

Typical meals

When you slow down and focus on the flavor and quality of your food, your idea of meals begins to change.

Breakfast is generally light. After all, you haven't been working up an appetite all night while you were sleeping. Breakfast might consist of coffee or tea with a croissant or tartine (toast) with a little butter and jam, or some yogurt and fresh fruit.

A normal lunch or dinner would be sensible, filling, and delicious, with a healthy balance of proteins, carbohydrates, and fats.

Some examples of this could be:

- A serving of fish or seafood atop a fresh salad

- A hearty soup with some nice, crusty bread

- Grilled fish, chicken, or a small steak with fresh roasted vegetables

- Some cheese and fresh bread, with a salad of tender greens

- An omelette, quiche, or scrambled eggs with fresh fruit or salad and bread

- A delicious Coq au vin (chicken stew cooked in wine) or Boeuf Bourguignon (beef stew) with some potatoes or noodles.

I hope this sounds delicious – it was meant to. These are all simple dishes, most of which can be prepared very quickly (except the stews, which have a longer cook time).

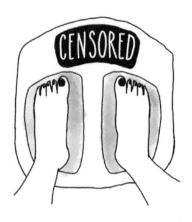

CHAPTER 9
IF YOU NEED TO LOSE WEIGHT

Following the 3 Factors and the French Metabolism Guidelines will allow you to maintain your optimum weight your entire life, enjoying delicious food on a regular basis and making little adjustments where needed to compensate for the occasional indulgence.

But what if you've got more than just a few pounds to lose, to get to that optimum weight?

Everything we've talked about before applies more than ever: you'll get yourself into a positive frame of mind, envisioning the goal and appreciating yourself and the changes you'll be seeing; you'll address your relationship with food, slow down, and appreciate the food you're eating; you'll prepare most of your meals at home with healthy, simple ingredients; and you'll incorporate movement into every day. But you'll need to be get a little more aggressive to get the excess weight off as quickly as possible while maintaining good health.

I won't tell you it's easy, but it is simple. Anything worth having is worth working for. And the adjustments you'll make are pretty painless.

Foods to focus on

It's much better to focus on what you should eat than what you shouldn't, wouldn't you agree?

When you need to lose weight, restrict your diet to only the following foods. The closer you adhere to this, the faster you'll lose the excess weight and sooner you'll be following a normal, sensible way of eating and enjoying the full cornucopia of foods you love.

Proteins – fish or seafood, beef, poultry, eggs, etc., prepared simply with a minimum of oil or butter and no sauces.

One of the best ways to prepare proteins is simply grilled with salt and pepper and a little oil. I recommend grapeseed oil for high-temperature grilling. It has a higher smoke point than olive oil, and will not leave a bitter taste.

Make a small investment in a good cast iron grill pan for grilling meats and even vegetables. It adds tremendous flavor without needing to add rich sauces or extra fats, and will be the best thirty or so bucks you've ever spent.

Vegetables – every color under the sun. Eat these fresh in a salad, in soups, grilled, or roasted in the oven with a little seasoning, garlic and olive oil.

Healthy fats – used in moderation (about a tablespoon a day). Use good oil, and buy it in relatively small bottles so it doesn't go rancid. Mostly your daily portion of fats will be used to season meats or vegetables, or for salad.

Only have one piece of fruit per day, which you may want to have with yogurt or in a smoothie for breakfast, or eaten later as a late afternoon snack or dessert.

Restrict dairy to yogurt, and buy plain, full-fat yogurt. Yogurt is filling and a great source of probiotics. If you find plain yogurt too sour for your taste, sweeten it up a bit with some fresh fruit and/or a little drizzle of honey (about ½ a teaspoon should do the trick). Don't succumb to the fruit-flavored or non-fat versions of yogurt; both tend to be highly processed and contain excessive amounts of sugar.

Water, water, and more water – consuming water is a natural appetite suppressant, and it allows your body to eliminate the unwanted goo. Make sure to get your daily quota – half your body weight in ounces. You can drink tea and coffee too, of course, but no fruity drinks, soda, or diet soda.

Keep preparing essentially the same delicious meals you normally would, just leaving off the breads and sweets and extras, until you've reached your desired weight.

Snacking

We've already discussed snacking, which is not a part of the French way of eating. But I'm bringing it up again here because it can be a huge pit-fall for those who need to lose weight, and may be one of the key reasons you're overweight.

The French way of eating includes ample food at mealtime, and no snacking. Allowing yourself to eat between meals keeps you focused on food throughout the day keeps a constant stream of insulin, a fat-producing hormone, circulating through the body; and it keeps your mind on food throughout the day.

If you find yourself wanting to snack between meals out of habit, well, that's when your passion comes into play. Remind yourself that you are creating a new metabolism, and besides, soon (within a few hours) you will have a meal. It takes just a few weeks to break a habit, and very soon you'll find you aren't foraging for snacks between meals.

If you feel you just must have something between meals, try having a cup of your favorite tea, or a small (not heaping) teaspoon of nut butter which you'll lick like a lollipop, or maybe 3 or 4 olives (which are great for killing sugar cravings).

I don't keep snacks in the house, because, like the French, I don't snack. This works great, because you can't eat what you don't have.

And remember especially, after dinner the kitchen is closed.

So why not just go keto?

This may sound close to keto, with the exception of the dairy and fruit. So why not just go keto?

Well, you could, but here's my problems with the ketogenic diet:

- Medical professionals do not agree that it is a healthy way to eat,

- It relies on excessive amounts of fat and protein which can be hard on the body,

- It relies on maintaining a certain chemistry (ketosis), in order to be effective. If you go wrong, slip up, or miscalculate, the chemistry is destroyed and all you've done is eaten a lot of fat and protein, which will sabotage what you're trying to accomplish.

- And most of all, it's not sustainable and doesn't address your relationship with food and your eating behavior. So unless you actually love eating that way and plan to do so for the rest of your life, you will very likely gain everything back when you return to your "normal" way of eating.

That said, if it works well for you and your lifestyle, go for it. But apply the guidelines, learning to pace yourself, not over-eating, and adjusting your relationship with food. That way, you'll set yourself up for success if and when you do return to a less restrictive way of eating.

There's really no need to go to extremes, which you may have difficulty sticking with. Just enjoy the bounty of foods listed above in reasonable proportions, applying the guidelines, and keep at it until you've achieved your goal. By following the basic factors and guidelines, temporarily reducing the dairy and fats, getting plenty of water, and leaving off the sugar and bread, you will see an immediate and steady weight loss.

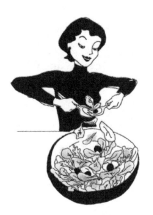

CHAPTER 10
KITCHEN STAPLES, MEAL SUGGESTIONS,
AND SIMPLE RECIPES

We all have our superpowers. Mine, besides knowing what day something I'm expecting will arrive in the mail and making parking spots materialize, is being able to throw a meal together when there's "nothing in the house", even if guests show up unexpectedly.

By now it should come as no surprise that many of my favorite movies are either about food or France, and if they're about food *and* France ... heaven. Such is the case with "The Hundred-Foot Journey".

What especially inspired me was the scene where Marguerite

(Charlotte Le Bon) treats Hassan (Manish Dayal) and family, to a simple feast from the family larder. Oh. My. God.

While you, like me, may not live where you can just pluck a few fresh eggs out from under a chicken's ass or forage mushrooms from the forest, still there are many amazing dishes you can prepare at a moments' notice just by keeping a few basics in the house.

For the pantry

Jarred sundried tomatoes
Canned or jarred artichoke hearts
Kalamata olives
Cornichon (little French pickles)
San Marzano whole tomatoes
Chicken broth
Dried lentils
Quinoa
Canned beans (garbanzos, pintos, black)
Fruit spread (my favorites are Dalmatia fig spread and Bon Maman preserves)
Dried spices (oregano, thyme, cinnamon, cumin, ginger, basil, parsley, red chili flakes)
Salt and pepper
Flour
Sugar
Onions (last 1 month on the counter or 1-2 months in the fridge)
Garlic (lasts 3-6 months on the counter)
Dried pasta (linguini and bowtie are my favorites)
Olive oil
Grapeseed or avocado oil (for high-heat cooking)
Crackers or flatbread

For the fridge

Eggs (last 3-5 weeks in the fridge)
Butter (lasts about a month in the fridge)
Lemons (last in the fridge for 2-4 months)
Cheeses (hard cheese lasts about 2-4 months, semi-hard cheeses last 1-2 months, soft cheeses last 1-2 weeks, so choose accordingly)
Fresh fruits and vegetables, which you'll consume in a few days

For the freezer

Meat, fish, chicken (fish is especially good because it thaws quickly, in case you forget to put something out)
Shrimp (get raw, not cooked – you can't cook cooked shrimp)
Fruits
Puff pastry

Here are some French and some not-so-French suggestions for simple daily meals. It's by no means a guide to what you must eat, but if you're not accustomed to preparing meals at home, it will get you started.

* Indicates recipe below

Breakfast

Yogurt Bowl*

Breakfast Smoothie*

French Scrambled Eggs* and toast

Lunches and Dinners

Poached eggs* on Avocado Toast*

The Daily Salad*

Hearty chicken soup*

Lentil soup*

Delicious (Believe it or Not) Kale Salad*

Crispy Skin Salmon* with Charred Broccoli*

Best-Ever Turkey Burger*

Frittata*

Any fresh, hearty soup with crusty bread

Any fresh salad with some grilled chicken, scallops or other protein

Any grilled meat* with any roasted vegetable*

Yogurt Bowl

This is kind of a no-brainer.

The most important thing is using organic, plain, full-fat yogurt.

Add to that fresh fruit in season (think berries in the summer, pomegranate and persimmon in the winter), or thaw some organic, flash-frozen fruits.

Add some nuts and seeds and maybe a little sprinkling of granola for a little crunch, and a little drizzle of honey if you need some extra sweetness.

Smoothie

The basic smoothie is half a banana, a handful of spinach, a frozen or fresh fruit such as strawberries, blueberries, mango, or pineapple (whatever you like), and a cup of unsweetened almond milk.

To get a little fancy and pack in some extra nutrients, you can add any combination of:

- A tablespoon of coconut oil (use virgin coconut oil if you like the flavor of coconuts, regular if you don't),
- A tablespoon of chia seeds,
- A tablespoon of ground flax seeds,
- Good quality protein powder,
- Collagen powder,
- A half teaspoon of matcha green tea.

French Scrambled Eggs

This is not your mama's scrambled eggs, unless your mama is from France.

The secret to these eggs is very low heat and lots of stirring.

Prep time: About 10 minutes
Serves 2

4 large eggs

1 T butter

1 T crème fraiche (optional)

Salt to taste

Crack the eggs into a bowl, add a pinch of sea salt, and use a whisk to beat into a frenzy. Yolks and whites should be fully incorporated.

Melt the butter in a nonstick skillet over low heat. Add the eggs and immediately start to scramble, keeping the eggs moving, until small curds start to form.

Eggs should be cooked very slowly over very low heat. If they start to cook too fast and larger curds start to form, simply remove the pan from the heat for a few seconds to slow it down.

When eggs are about half-way set, add about a tablespoon of crème fraiche and continue stirring, incorporating the crème fraiche into the eggs.

Eggs are done when they are still very moist but no longer runny.

Season to taste with salt and pepper.

Poached Eggs

I've made everything from croissants to standing rib roast, but I was completely intimidated by poached eggs until I found this method by Alton Brown.

Prep time: 5 minutes
Serves 2

4 large eggs

1 T distilled vinegar

Pinch of salt

Water

Bring about 2" of water to a gentle boil in a saucepan appropriately sized for the number of eggs you'll be poaching. (I generally use my 10" skillet for poaching 4 eggs.) Add about a tablespoon of distilled vinegar, and a good pinch of salt.

Break the eggs one by one into a small dish, and gently lower each egg into the gently boiling water.

When the eggs are in the water, turn off the burner, cover with a lid, and let them poach. No peeking – just wait and trust, and set the timer for 4 minutes. Then gently lift your perfectly poached eggs out of the water with a slotted spoon.

Avocado Toast

Sure, you can just slap some avocado on a toast, but we can do better than that.

The measurements don't need to be precise, you can just eyeball it. Leave out the jalapeno if you don't particularly want it spicy.

Prep time: About 10 minutes
Servings: 2

Basic guacamole:

1 Fresh, ripe avocado

1 T finely minced red onion

1 t finely minced garlic

1 T finely minced jalapeno (seeds and ribs removed)

1 T chopped cilantro

Juice of half a lemon

Salt to taste

Combine all ingredients in a small bowl and squish it up with a fork, leaving it a little lumpy.

Spread on toast and eat it as-is, or top it with one of your perfectly poached eggs with a little sea salt and pepper.

The Daily Salad

I have some version of this salad pretty much every day, hence the name.

I make my salads upside down. Most people make salads by putting a big gob of greens in the bowl and chopping up "stuff" to throw on top. By chopping up the "stuff" and then adding the greens, the stuff-to-greens ratio is better. Plus when you toss it, the "stuff" gets distributed better and doesn't wind up on the bottom.

Combine as many as you want of the following ingredients that are seasonally fresh and appeal to you – you can't go wrong.

Greens:

Arugula
Spring mix
Endive
Radicchio
Spinach

Proteins:

Grilled chicken
Toasted chili garbanzos*
Feta
Goat cheese
Pine nuts
Walnuts

Extras:

Cherry tomatoes

Red, green and yellow bell pepper
Kalamata olives
Red onion
Cucumber
Avocado
Pomegranate seeds
Strawberries

For the dressing

2 T olive oil
2-3 cloves garlic, pressed in a garlic press
Juice of ½ lemon
Pinch of salt

Whisk ingredients together and you're done.

For the Toasted Chili Garbanzos

Drain and rinse 1 can of garbanzo beans. Either do this an hour or so ahead of preparing, or place on a paper towel to dry.

Heat a cast iron skillet on high with about a tablespoon of oil.

Add the garbanzos and reduce heat to medium.

Sprinkle with a pinch of salt and some dried chili powder to taste (about a tablespoon), and allow them to toast until they start to pop and brown slightly.

Hearty Chicken Soup

For me, this is the winter equivalent to a salad. Think about it, you have a lean protein and a whole lot of fresh vegetables, but instead of raw and crunchy they're soft and warm with all those wonderful nutrients steeped into a flavorful broth.

In the cooler months I almost always have a pot of this (or some other soup) in the fridge. It's a great quick lunch or dinner.

The vegetables I've listed are the ones I always add, but it's also a great way to use up bits of veggies you haven't had a chance to cook, like that last zucchini or piece of broccoli that's left hanging out in the fridge.

Prep time: About 30 minutes
Cook time: About an hour
Serves: 4-6, with leftovers

1 whole chicken or chicken parts (I prefer skinless, boneless thighs)

Water

1 T salt

1 medium onion, chopped

4 or more (up to you) cloves of garlic, chopped

4-5 stalks of celery, sliced crosswise

4-5 carrots, sliced into coins

½ head of cabbage, chopped

Thumb-sized piece of fresh ginger, grated

1-2 T turmeric

1 T cumin

1 T dried thyme

1 T dried oregano

½ lemon

Salt and pepper

If using a whole chicken, rinse and remove the giblets, if included. Place the whole chicken or chicken parts in a large soup pot, with enough salted water to cover it. Bring to a boil, reduce heat and cover, and continue to simmer for about 20 minutes, until the thigh separates easily (for a whole chicken) and juices are clear.

While chicken is boiling, prepare the vegetables. Roughly chop into uniform, bite-sized pieces.

Remove the chicken from the pot into a large bowl, and let stand for about 10 minutes to cool slightly. Meanwhile, place the chopped vegetables in the broth and add seasonings to taste. Let this simmer while you prepare the chicken.

Remove skin and bones, if any, from the chicken, and cut into bite-sized pieces. Add the cut-up chicken back to the pot and continue to simmer another 30 minutes or so, tasting and adjusting seasonings.

Lentil Soup

This is the other soup that's in the fridge when the chicken soup isn't in the fridge.

Prep time: About 20 minutes
Cook time: About an hour
Serves: 4-6, with leftovers

1 lb dried lentils, well rinsed

2 T olive oil

1 medium onion, chopped

4 or more (up to you) cloves of garlic, chopped

4-5 stalks of celery, sliced crosswise

4-5 carrots, sliced into coins

1 bunch of kale, chopped into bite-sized pieces

1 – 2 qt. chicken stock

1 T dried thyme

1 T dried oregano

1T turmeric

1t ground cumin

Additional seasonings to taste (cardamom, nutmeg, cayenne)

1T salt

Place the olive oil, onions, garlic, celery and carrots in a soup pot over medium heat, and add the dry seasonings to "toast" the seasonings while you soften the vegetables.

Add 1 qt. chicken stock and the dried lentils. Bring to a boil and simmer about 45 minutes, adjusting seasoning. Add additional chicken stock or water as needed to desired consistency. Soup is done when lentils and veggies are completely tender.

For a variation and to add creaminess and an Indian flavor, stir in a can of coconut milk and some fresh grated ginger. Simmer another 5 minutes.

Delicious (Believe it or Not) Kale Salad

There are a lot of people who would tell you that the words "delicious" and "kale" do not belong in the same sentence. To those people I ask, "are you massaging your kale?"

Raw kale, chopped up and placed in a bowl is about as appealing as eating a toilet paper roll. Here's the trick: drizzle a half tablespoon or so of olive oil over it, add a small pinch of sea salt, and massage it like it's your best friend. Squeeze the heck out of it until it's reduced in volume by about one-third and has a soft, chewable texture.

From here, you have options –

Add a sweet element – some pomegranate seeds, golden raisins, grapefruit sections or dried cranberries

Add a crunch element – some slivered almonds, walnut pieces or toasted pine nuts (my favorite)

Add a couple ounces of feta, crumbled

Other great additions – diced avocado, slivers of red onion, Kalamata olives, cucumber

Dress with lemon juice and a little more olive oil if desired. Toss and be amazed.

By the way, I always recommend buying feta in a block and crumbling it yourself – it's a lot less expensive than the pre-crumbled one, to which stabilizers have been added to keep it crumbled. And buy the full-fat version – food should be eaten in its native, less processed state.

Crispy Skin Salmon

Wild caught or farm raised? It's quite a controversy, but here's what I can tell you: studies have shown that both are pretty equal in terms of Omega 3's.

Personally, I really prefer farm raised. It is a milder, fattier fish, and fat is delicious. I buy from a reputable market that sources their aquaculture (farmed fish) responsibly and does not allow antibiotics, growth hormones, or genetic modification. And I think that's about the best you can do.

Prep time: 5 minutes
Cook time: 10-15 minutes
Serves 2

About ¾ lb. piece of salmon, skin on

Grapeseed oil

Salt and Pepper

For 2 servings, cut an approximately 8 – 12 oz. piece of salmon crosswise into 2 pieces.

Make 2 or 3 scores across the skin with a sharp knife. This will allow you to get seasoning in the skin and also will prevent the fish from curling.

Season with salt, rubbing sea salt into the scores, and black pepper if desired.

Heat a cast iron skillet over high heat, and add a tablespoon or two of grapeseed oil – enough to coat the pan. (FYI, for years I used olive oil. However grapeseed oil has a much higher smoke point and will not give a bitter taste to the fish.)

When the pan is almost smoking hot, place the fish skin side down in the pan. Reduce temperature to medium high and cook about 2 minutes, until the skin no longer sticks to the pan and is brown and crisp.

Gently turn the fish once, cooking another 2 or 3 minutes until fish is lightly browned and cooked through to desired doneness. If the piece of fish you've chosen is quite thick, pop the pan in a 350 degree oven for about 5 or 10 minutes to finish.

Serve skin side up. If you're serving with a sauce, serve the sauce under the fish, not on top, to preserve the crispy skin.

Charred Broccoli

If you haven't caught on yet, I love cooking in cast iron. The original non-stick cookware, it imparts nutrients and more flavor than you can imagine into your food. Plus nothing else gets the crust or char that you can get with cast iron.

Prep time: 5 minutes
Cook time: About 5 minutes
Serves 2

1 head of broccoli

3-4 cloves of garlic

Grapeseed oil

Cut the head of broccoli into uniform pieces, so that pieces are not terribly thick and there is good surface area.

Heat a cast iron skillet coated well with grapeseed oil over medium-high heat. Add the broccoli and stir, allowing pieces to get slightly charred but not burnt.

After about 2 minutes, add the garlic to the pan and cook another 3 or 4 minutes until broccoli is nicely charred and slightly tender, and garlic is browned.

Best Ever Turkey Burgers

I love a good hunk of meat on a bun, but we don't eat a lot of red meat at our house. Turkey burgers are a great alternative for a burger night.

Turkey burgers can be bland and dry and not unlike cardboard. These burgers are juicy and teeming with flavor, with hints of Indian spices. I came up with this recipe because it just felt right, and it turned out to be the best turkey burger I'd ever eaten.

The proportions are not rocket surgery – the tablespoon of sriracha makes it mild to medium-spicy, so adjust that along with the other seasonings according to you taste.

Prep time: About 10 minutes
Cook time: About 10 minutes
Serves 4

1 lb. ground turkey (I prefer dark meat, but your choice)

2 cloves of finely minced garlic (about a tablespoon)

¼ of a small apple, grated

2 T finely minced red onion

1 knuckle-sized piece (about a tablespoon) fresh ginger, grated

½ t ground cumin

1 t Kosher salt

¼ t freshly ground black pepper

1 T Sriracha sauce

A squeeze of fresh lemon

Place everything in a bowl and squish together, fully incorporating all ingredients. The mixture is quite moist so you will not be able to handle it a great deal, but it firms up when you cook it.

Divide into 4 portions and shape into patties (you'll want them to be fairly thin since they will be cooked through – no rare turkey).

Heat a skillet (preferably cast iron, of course) coated with a little grapeseed oil over medium high heat. When the skillet is very hot, carefully place the patties.

Reduce heat to medium and cook about 3-4 minutes on each side. The outside should be nicely carmelized and inside should no longer be pink (juices should be clear).

Serve on a toasted whole grain bread or bun (or skip the bun), with sliced avocado, arugula, mayonnaise and mustard

Frittata

Frittata is a great, simple main course for lunch, brunch or dinner, and you can whip it up in no time. Serve it with a little side salad and some crusty bread for a delicious "peasant's feast".

Prep time: 10 minutes

Cook time: 15 minutes

Serves 4-6

6 large eggs
¼ cup light or heavy cream
1 t sea salt
¼ t freshly ground pepper
1 T olive oil
½ small onion
2-3 cloves of garlic
About a cup of shredded cheese (Gruyere, Fontina, Parmesan) or crumbled Feta

Anything you have on hand – bacon, ham, leftover chicken, sundried tomatoes, artichoke hearts (well drained), spinach, tomatoes, sliced potatoes, etc.

Heat the oven to 400 degrees F.

Whisk the eggs and cream, add salt and pepper, and set aside.

If using bacon, cook it first in a cast iron or oven safe non-stick skillet. Remove from the pan and drain off all but about 2 teaspoons of the fat. If you're not using bacon, add about 1 tablespoon of olive oil to the pan.

Saute the onion, garlic, and any other extras you'll be using until tender, about 3-5 minutes. Crumble the bacon, if using, and add it back in.

Pour the egg mixture into the skillet. Tilt the pan or lightly use a rubber spatula to help distribute the eggs evenly over the vegetables, being careful not to avoid scraping the bottom of the pan.

Add the cheese, again lightly using a rubber spatula and not scraping the bottom. Cook over medium heat about 2 minutes, until eggs begin to set around the edges.

Pop it in the oven for about 10 minutes until the eggs are set (insert a knife to check for doneness).

Frittata can be served warm, room temperature, or even cold depending on the ingredients.

Grilled steak or chicken breast

Honestly, simple is best. Using the cast iron grill pan gives amazing flavor to the meat. Plus if you're serving with any sauce or dressing, the flavors will not conflict.

Prep time: 2 minutes
Cook time: 10 minutes
Serves 2

2 Rib eye, filet or cut of your choice of steak, or chicken breast sliced lengthwise

Grapeseed oil

Salt and pepper

Heat a grill pan to almost smoking hot.

Season meat with salt and pepper and rub with grapeseed oil – nothing else.

Reduce heat to medium high and cook steak to desired doneness, or cook chicken until juices run clear.

Allow the meat to rest at least 10 minutes before slicing, to retain juices.

When I grill chicken, I always cook extra to use in a future salad. Just refrigerate and slice when ready – warm it in a skillet with a little olive oil or enjoy cold.

Roasted Brussels Sprouts (or any roasted vegetable)

Almost any vegetable tastes amazing when roasted. Because you're not cooking in water or excessive oil, roasting intensifies the flavor and keeps all the nutrients inside the vegetable.

Prep time: 5-10 minutes
Cook time: About 20 minutes
Serves about 4

1 lb. Brussels sprouts (or other dense vegetable)

3 – 4 cloves of garlic, chopped

Olive oil

Salt and pepper

Preheat oven to 425 degrees.

Slice Brussels sprouts in half. If using other types of vegetable, prepare to uniform thickness (whether sliced or cubed) so that cooking time will be even. Sprinkle with salt and pepper, and coat with olive oil.

Place in a single layer on a foil-lined sheet tray (you'll thank me when it's time to clean up) and roast in the oven for about 10 minutes.

After about 10 minutes, stir or turn the vegetables and sprinkle with the chopped garlic. Continue roasting about another 10 minutes, or until vegetables are brown and tender, stirring again if needed.

Serve as-is or drizzle with a little dense Balsamic vinegar.

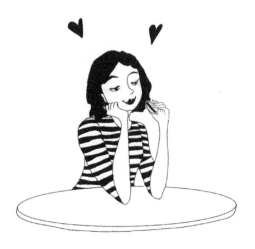

CHAPTER 11
YOUR FINAL FRENCH METABOLISM GUIDELINE

I've saved one important thing for last:

> *French Metabolism Guideline – Always Consider the Pleasure Factor*

In the French way of life, the pleasure factor is a consideration in anything you do. Guilt is not.

What's more pleasurable right now? Is it going ahead and enjoying that special dessert? Or is it passing something up because you know you're on your way to being 10, 20 or more pounds slimmer, knowing that, after all, you can always have it later? The answer can be different at different times, depending on the circumstances.

If you're on a quest to lose weight, I want to encourage you to delay the gratification of special treats until you've made some significant headway. It will be more rewarding to see the change in fit of your clothes, or the lower number on the scale, than that 10 minutes of indulgence. Nothing is more encouraging than progress.

Either way, it's your choice, and you win.

Remember, no matter what, where, or how you're eating, the 3 Factors and the French Metabolism Guidelines play a role. They provide the means of enjoying what you want, when you want, in a healthy, moderate and sustainable way.

À ton bel avenir – to your beautiful future.

FRENCH METABOLISM CHEAT SHEET

The 3 Factors that Create the French Metabolism

Your Relationship With Food
The Quality of Food
Movement (Exercise)

French Metabolism Guidelines

Create a positive self-image, and wear it with confidence
Put. The fork. Down.
Don't eat if you're not hungry, and when you're full, stop eating
It's okay to feel a little hungry
Eat all you need *to eat, not all you* can *eat*
Eat at meal times, and don't skip meals
Drink plenty of water
After dinner, the kitchen is closed
Monitor. And Moderate
Get enough sleep
Avoid highly processed foods
Eat at home
Buy the best food you can
Buy local and seasonal
Don't eat food that doesn't taste good
Eat your veggies
Move every day
Walk whenever and wherever you can
Stay active throughout the day
Always consider the pleasure factor

WHAT'S NEXT?

Subscribe to my blog, KelleyPom.com, for inspiration on living a beautiful French life, no matter where you are.

Join our community on Facebook for tips and recipes, support and inspiration.

https://www.facebook.com/kelleypom/

Need more help or want more guidance to achieve your goals?
Email me for one-on-one coaching
Kelley@SoFreakingFrench.com

KELLEY POM

ABOUT THE AUTHOR

Kelley Pom has received awards in journalist writing and prose, and has published columns in several publications. She's been writing her blog, SoFreakingFrench.com, since 2016.

Having been raised in the very shallow end of the gene pool, and creating a life which can only be described as artistic and elegant, Kelley is steadfast in the belief that anyone from anywhere can create a beautiful life. She's on a mission to share the art of living.

This is Kelley's first book.

Made in the USA
Monee, IL
29 September 2021

79062082R00059